THE

GREEN

SMOOTHIE FIX

The Ultimate Smoothie Cleanse to
Maximize Your Health and Well-being

J.C. Collins

ISBN-10: 1502458934
ISBN-13: 978- 1502458933

DEDICATION

This book is dedicated to those in search of proven methods to maximize your health with the help of the green smoothie cleanse.

CONTENTS

INTRODUCTION

Green smoothies are a delicious way to improve the overall health of your body, while also getting rid of unwanted toxins. They are made up of fruits, greens, and water, which makes them fast and easy to prepare. Many people are afraid to try them because they do not like the taste of greens, but, to tell the truth, you can barely taste the greens in the smoothie.

Consuming green smoothies on a regular basis offers a host of different health benefits. One blender full of green smoothies can provide as many as eight servings of fruits and vegetables per day. This is why they should be incorporated into any diet plan.

CHAPTER 1 – THE TRUTH ABOUT CLEANSING

Cleansing is always associated with the words detoxification, weight loss, diet, juicing, Gwyneth Paltrow and sometimes even enema! While the true sense of the term cleansing has been obscured by media hype, outright wrong understanding of human biology and opportunists who take advantage of a new fad to make more money, it is best to stick with your literal understanding of the word – Cleansing is cleansing. End of story.

If you want to be more technical about it, cleansing is choosing a particular time where all the bad stuff you have been consuming all your life will be briefly replaced by a nutrient and antioxidant rich substitute. This will serve to rejuvenate your cells and give you energy so that you can live a healthier life.

Unfortunately, people give so many wrong, exaggerated, almost ludicrous annotations to cleansing. Let us bust some myths first before we proceed:

Myth #1: Cleansing involves colon cleansing

There is no medical basis whatsoever that periodic flushing the colon will help you get rid of diseases. This assumption was fueled by the misunderstanding that fecal matter can get impacted for years in the colon which can cause many diseases. The truth is, eating a diet rich in fiber will suffice. Frequent flushing of the colon may disrupt the normal balance between the good and bad bacterial populations which can cause more harm than good.

The truth:

The only way to make things easier for the colon is to drink plenty of water, eat a lot of fiber-rich foods and encourage beneficial bacteria to proliferate through probiotics. With the right ingredients, a green smoothie can accomplish all of these.

Myth #2: Most illnesses are caused by "toxins" and you need to detoxify

Most people use fear to sell ideas and most of the time, products. The fear of vague "toxins" is one of the main driving forces why cleansing and detoxification have become so popular. Proponents go as far as to claim that people will get rid of cancers, diabetes and a host of other unrelated diseases if they always detoxify. The premise here is that every day, your body is bombarded by "toxins" that eventually build-up on your body over time to cause health problems. Some claim that purging out these toxins will cure you of all your diseases.

Toxins are described as exogenous or endogenous in origin. Endogenous toxins are toxins that your cells constantly produce as a by-product of normal cell metabolism. Exogenous toxins are those toxins that come from the environment, particularly in food, beverages and even pollutants. To think that the body needs help on getting rid of these toxins is quite absurd. Unless you have kidney or liver problems, the body is fairly capable of cleaning and purging itself of these "toxins". The term detoxification itself has been twisted. In reality, detoxification pertains to a medical procedure that is done on poisoned patients using specialized equipment and scientific procedures.

The Truth:

Environmental pollutants such as lead, mercury and volatile organic compounds are proven to have bad effects to your health. There are also carcinogenic compounds that can really induce cell mutation and cause cancer as well as free-radicals that can destroy your cells (and accelerate aging!) through oxidative stress.

These substances can come from pesticide residues left from conventionally produced crops, house cleaning agents and even everyday items that you use. HOWEVER, we did not evolved as the apex species of planet earth if these mere substances can stop us! As was mentioned, the body is fairly capable of protecting itself not just from bacteria, viruses and parasites but also from these harmful substances.

To try to shun from the above substances is futile. For example, chronic exposure to radiation from nuclear plants, x-ray and ultraviolet rays are found to have adverse health effects. The problem What cleansing does is to improve your body's capability to protect itself by temporarily withdrawing from bad foods and stress and drinking highly nutritious green smoothies – Cleansing is not a mechanical/chemical process of excreting "toxins", it is a way to strengthen the body to better cope with these "toxins".

Myth #3: Cleansing will definitely make you lose weight

Cleansing is not a diet fad; it is a way of life. Losing some pounds is only a good "side effect" of healthier living. People sell the idea that cleansing fixes everything: from cancers, heart diseases, diabetes to obesity. The process of weight loss will largely depend on eating the right types of food, the amount of exercise, genetics and lastly your overall health condition; while juicing diets can really trim down fats since you will starve yourself (juices may be highly nutritious but they contain no fiber, fat or protein). Pounds lost will surely creep back once one finishes the diet and revert to his/her old ways of unhealthy eating.

The Truth:

As you will read later on, green smoothie cleansing will be so healthy, your body will lose some extra pounds along the way. This is because you will be barred from eating processed foods particularly those nasty refined carbohydrates. If you indeed lost some weight, then it only means that your body has put on some extra pounds that can be "burned" through exercise and refraining from processed foods.

Cleansing is pampering your whole body by trying to get rid of all the bad stuff and shifting to a high fiber, high nutrient diet for a time. It gives your body a reset or fresh start. For some people, the effects will be seen right away and many give anecdotal stories about how their skin glowed, how they slept better, how stronger they become, how they lost this amount of pounds and how they generally felt better. Theoretically, these effects are possible especially if your smoothie is really healthy.

If you do not experience these effects, however, then do not be disturbed. Cleansing is just cleansing. It is not meant to be a fix-all-solution to all your problems. Sometimes, it may even take more "sips" of green smoothies to actually feel the effects. But think about this: The mere fact that you are doing your body a favor by drinking a super nutritious drink is enough reason to feel happy and contented; this is true for most people. Once you see the good effects of what cleansing will do for you, this may even be the start of living a healthier lifestyle.

J.C. Collins

CHAPTER 2 – HOW DO I CLEANSE?

Cleansing involves picking a period of time when you will cut down on processed foods, meat (optional), refined carbohydrates, junk food, nicotine and alcohol. Only nutritious foods such as green salads and organic foods are allowed. Drugs are only allowed if they are prescribed by your doctor (especially maintenance drugs). Sleep must not also be less than 8 hours so it is important to abstain from activities that promote sleep-skipping.

A positive attitude must ideally be adopted at all times during cleanse days/weeks so it is also preferable if you can distance yourself away from things that trigger stress. Some people also take the opportunity cleanse days provide to exercise but it is best to avoid strenuous physical activities.

Cleanses can be as short as 1 day to as long as 7 days. The choice lies on what is more convenient for you but for maximum results, a 7-day cleanse is recommended. As long as you carefully follow the instructions, however, even a 1-day cleanse can provide you with the rejuvenation your body needs. By the time that you are finished cleansing, your body is ready to take on new challenges

Why only eat healthy foods?

The idea is, as you are eating more healthily (as much as possible, no junk foods, processed foods and refined carbohydrates) and drinking large amounts of highly nutritious green smoothies, the nutrients will be more readily integrated into your body and you feel stronger and refreshed. The problem with "eating healthily" is that most people misconstrue it as deprivation and veggie overload. Eating healthily is about making informed choices on the foods that you eat.

You should always ask yourself if the food that you eat is really good for you (chapter 3 can actually help you with that). It is important not to deprive yourself during cleansing. Some people advocate that only smoothies or juices should touch your gut during cleanse days, as in no food for the whole duration! The problem with this is some people will have mood swings, be irritated or worse, fall into depression.

Deprived people also have a bigger chance of binging on unhealthy foods like cakes, doughnuts and pastries that are full of refined carbohydrates as well as doing some rebound eating after a diet. To prevent this, try to eat the right foods in the right amounts during cleansing and do not push yourself too hard. If you feel too attached to an unhealthy snack, try to reduce its consumption first up to what is tolerable for you and work towards gradually diminishing if not eliminating it from your normal diet.

Why sleep is important?

By sleeping at least 8 hours and shying away from stress, your body's energy will be shifted to facilitate cell repair and regeneration as well as facilitating "cleaning" of free radicals through antioxidants. The crucial part here is to relax and minimize stress during cleanse days so that you can maximize sleep. It is said that the most regenerative sleep happens between 10pm to 2am. As was pointed out in chapter 1, the body is fairly equipped to fight off "toxins" and free radicals that destroy cells.

One such "cleaning equipment" is the hormone called melatonin, which is at peak production between 10pm to 2am during sleep. People who wake up or stay awake till 10pm has impaired natural free radical removal so staying away from stressful activities and limiting the use of the computer, particularly social media during bedtime is profoundly recommended. Sleep is also the time when the brain consolidates memory, the muscles are repaired and hormones valuable to regulating appetite is released. Restorative sleep during cleanse days will definitely go far when resilience is concerned.

Why do you need positivity?

The mind and body cannot be separated. What the mind can conceive, the body will do everything to fulfill. The power of visualizing positive thoughts is now being recognized as an important pillar in health and well-being even if the exact mechanisms of how it does so are not clearly understood. Positive thoughts do not just put a happy smile on your face, according to research, it can increase your life span, aid your immune system, lower depression and reduce the chance of death from cardiovascular diseases.

Positive thinking will also help you cope during cleansing. As you are undergoing cleansing, focus on the positive feelings of relaxation that you will feel. After the cleansing, be observant of the positive changes that happened. Did somebody ask you why your skin was glowing? Did you lose weight? Did you feel more relaxed during times when normally you would succumb to stress? Did you sleep better? Did you feel more energetic?

Remember that some of these changes will become more apparent after a longer cleansing period and after a series of cleanses. This will help you control rebound eating after cleansing. People also have a tendency to party heavily (and overindulge on alcohol) after cleanse periods.

To Exercise or Not to Exercise

Due to lack of time, cleanse days are also utilized by some people to exercise and work out. There is a consensus that strenuous exercise must not be combined with fasting. Although the cleansing technique advocated by this book is far from fasting (you are encouraged to eat, but you should do so healthily), it is still best to refrain from exercises that have too much intensity and too long durations.

If you really want to exercise during cleansing, then putting dairy products in green smoothies and eating more meat during cleansing (remember that barring meat is optional) must be done to prevent muscle wasting and facilitate muscle repair. If done right and in moderate amounts, cleansing and exercise can provide you with energy to take on stress.

If you feel the following, then most likely you are in need of a cleansing period:

- You have trouble sleeping
- You are always tired despite having adequate amounts of sleep and regularly taking in high-

sugar and caffeinated drinks
- You suffer from bloating, constipation, diarrhea, or indigestion
- You would really like to get a break from stress
- You are hungry and binge on unhealthy food with prejudice
- You feel you are unhealthy

Of course, if you have these problems, there is always a chance that a more serious medical condition might have triggered these so pay attention to what your doctor will tell you. Remember, cleansing cannot promise you that you will get well from a serious disease or that it is the answer to obesity. What cleansing will do is to give you a fighting chance to shrug off stress and diseases by becoming stronger through a healthier lifestyle and high nutrient intake.

Is there something that I must know?

It is worthy to note that critics of green smoothie cleanse always point out a bad effect of green smoothies: oxalate build-up. According to them too much leafy greens can cause oxalate build-up in the kidney and may catalyze the formation of kidney stones. To be sure, always consult your physician to determine if you have any systemic diseases. The same is true for diabetics, especially those who have poor diabetes control. Too much fruit may cause an increase in blood sugar levels. Stabilize diabetes control first before trying any diet or cleanses.

J.C. Collins

CHAPTER 3 – HOW TO MAKE YOUR GREEN SMOOTHIE TRULY HEALTHY

Not all green smoothies are "blended" equally. The way you mix the ingredients as well as the ingredients themselves will determine if your green smoothie will really be healthy and suitable for cleansing. The more important question here is: What is healthy? It is obvious that everything that we know about the food we eat is in complete chaos.

For example, the hoax that is the food pyramid favored the consumption of carbohydrates over proteins and fats. This led to a great demand in refined carbohydrates and minimization of fat consumption.

30 years later, diabetes spread as if it was an epidemic. The view that we need that much carbohydrate is now being challenged not only by health buffs but by researchers as well. Knowing which is healthy and which is not will guide you in determining what to include in your

green smoothie blend.

Carbohydrates –

- Carbohydrates in a green smoothie will be supplied by fruits, sugar sweeteners and even starchy vegetables. Carbohydrates only become a menace if they are refined or processed. Processing removes the fiber and nutrients leaving only "naked" starches that are rapidly absorbed by the bloodstream that can cause a spike in your blood sugar level. Refined carbohydrates come into your diet as refined grains, sugar and their derivatives namely, white bread, pastries, white rice etc.

- It is now being recognized that constantly soaring blood sugar levels over long periods of time can lead to diabetes, obesity and even cardiovascular diseases. Too high sugar in your system can also induce more sugar cravings which can make you binge on sweets even more. Even if refined carbohydrates are the bad guys, great moderation is still needed on fruits and starchy vegetables.

Protein –

- People commonly put dairy products such as milk or cream in their smoothies and for a good reason: smoothies taste better with milk! Besides giving smoothies texture, dairy products are excellent sources of high quality protein. Proteins are used by the body as building blocks – proteins constitute hair, blood, part of the bones, skin, hair, muscles etc. That is justification enough to include protein rich ingredients in your smoothie blend. But did you know that protein can help in controlling your eating urges?

- Protein can induce a feeling of satiety longer than carbohydrates can which may aid in you in your weight loss battle. Other sources of protein that can be added to your smoothie blend are omega-3 egg yolks and protein powders.

Fats –

- Some of you might have cringed on the last line that read: egg yolks because (1) we are talking about raw eggs (maybe most of you are not fans of raw eggs) and (2) because it is also a known source of fat and cholesterol. Fats have been wrongly branded as the cause of most lifestyle diseases. As you may have read earlier, refined carbohydrates are in fact recognized as the culprits for those silent-killer diseases. While it is now recognized that there are good fats and bad fats, the assumption that saturated fats from eggs, dairy and some vegetable oils are bad for you is still a bit misleading.

- The only fats that should be avoided are the trans fats or the processed fats. This is found on margarine and most processed foods such as doughnuts, chips etc. (basically any processed food that has hydrogenated and partially hydrogenated oils). Studies have now shown that saturated fats may not be as bad as once thought.

- Like protein, an adequate portion of fat in the diet can also aid in maintaining a longer feeling of satiety that is beneficial on those who want to get in shape. Even if you eat adequate amounts of food containing vitamins A, D, E and K, you will not absorb much if you do not take them with fats. After all, these vitamins will not be called as fat soluble for nothing. And for the record, the omega-3 in organic eggs is considered to be a good fat – a fat that actually lowers cholesterol and has cardio-protective properties.

• If you still think that raw egg yolks are kind of gross, then did you know that some people even put colostrum in their smoothies? Yes we are talking about your mom's milk. Colostrum is also rich in saturated fat but it is now considered as a perfect food. After all, you grew because of it.

Now that you have the right foundation regarding most food groups, let us look at what should and should not be included in a healthy green smoothie:

Fruits –

• There are some people who dump fruits together with bad carbohydrates because of their sugar content. Indeed, it is true that some fruits can raise the blood sugar level especially if you gorge on it. To be safe, limit the fruits in a smoothie to at least 60% of the total ingredients. And as much as possible, use fruits that are grown organically without the use of pesticides. Remember, you want to cleanse, to be rid of things that should not be in your system. Pesticide residues are one of those.

• Fiber in fruits also helps facilitate good bowel movement and helps you fill full longer. Bananas are popular healthy additions to green smoothie as their flavor compliments that of vegetables, some say that adding bananas should be moderated as it may be too sweet (even if it contains fiber-bound carbohydrates).

- Avocados are excellent additions to any smoothie blend. It is essentially a complete food – it has fiber, some carbohydrates, protein and a decent amount of good fats. Some other fruit suggestions like papaya, apples and berries are all nutritious and delicious.

Vegetables –

- Like fruits, vegetables need to be as pesticide free as possible. Dark leafy greens like spinach are actually what give a green smoothie its distinct color. Dark leafy greens are loaded with fiber, antioxidants, vitamins and minerals. If fruits should contain roughly 60% of the green smoothie blend, then 40% should be filled in by vegetables.

- However, people who can tolerate the taste of vegetables tend to add more vegetables to their smoothie. Spinach for example, have high levels of antioxidants Vitamin E, A and C. It also contains anti-cancer and anti-inflammatory phytonutrients. Raw sprouts can also add B-vitamins as well as phytonutrients.

Dairy products –

- These include milk, yogurt, cream and kefir. Use unprocessed milk as much as possible. Do not use low-fat or fat free-yogurts. The processing that these yogurts undergo to be low-fat or fat-free removes fat at the expense of adding refined carbohydrates. Always stick to what is natural. Adding good amounts of dairy in a smoothie will not only improve its taste and texture but its fat and protein content will also fill you up more, minimizing your cravings. This can effectively make your green smoothie a one-bowl meal. Fermented dairy products such as yogurt and kefir contain probiotic bacteria which can aid in digestion and bowel movement.

Coconut milk, nut milks and hemp milks –

- If you are lactose intolerant or a vegan, dairy is obviously not an option as smoothie additions. Fortunately, there are many plant and nut-based milks that can be excellent and healthy milk substitutes. However, calling these milks as mere substitutes is quite belittling for these milks are excellent sources of protein and good fats. If you do not like coconut milk, there are plenty of nut milk options to choose from such as almond milk, walnut milk, cashew milk, hazelnut milk etc. If you are allergic to these nuts, then you can try hemp milk which has a good amount of good fats.

Additional protein sources –

- If you are still not contended with the protein from dairy or you are trying to bulk-up muscles, you can try to add other protein sources. The simplest and most basic are protein powders. Flavored protein powders can also add some excitement to your smoothie. If you want it more natural, omega-3 egg yolks are great options as these can also add texture and provide a healthy dose of good fats to your smoothie. Unprocessed peanut butters are also good protein sources that can add a nutty flavor to your smoothie.

Sweeteners –

- This largely depends on your taste. Some can tolerate drinking green smoothies without adding any sweeteners other than fruits while some like their smoothies sweet. Regular sugar is only an option if you will only put small amounts. If you want your smoothie to be sweeter, then other sweeteners such as organic honey and stevia are healthier options. If you do not have any issues with sugar substitutes, you may use them if you want to. Agave sugar is not as good as most people think so it is not included in the list.

Thinners –

- Clean water is the cheapest thinner to use and all people obviously do not have any issues or allergies associated with it. If you are a little bored with water, healthier alternatives such as coconut water and extra virgin coconut oil can be used. Coconut water generally has a lot of potassium which makes it excellent for people who want to replenish ions lost in exercise. It also contains some anti-cancer and anti-aging factors as well as the immune system boosting lauric acid.

- Up to 2 tablespoons of extra virgin coconut oil can be added to a green smoothie so you can benefit from its immune boosting factor (it has more lauric acid than coconut water) and Alzheimer's disease protecting functions. Coconut oil is fat so it can help you feel more sated and it is also a rich source of good fats that can protect your heart.

Spices –

- Spices not only add zest to your smoothie, they are also excellent sources of nutrients beneficial during cleansing. The most common spices are ginger, mint, cayenne, cinnamon and pure vanilla extract. Ginger, in particular has anti-inflammatory properties that can ease muscle and joint pains after an exercise while its pro-digestive properties make it ideal for cleansing. Some people even drink ginger tea during their cleansing days in addition to green smoothies. Cinnamon, specifically ceylon cinnamon has blood sugar regulating properties that may be beneficial for diabetics and prediabetics. Only ceylon cinnamon is proven to have this effect however.

Tips to Get Full Benefits of Smoothies

Imagine all of these nutrients combined in one delicious drink – the green smoothie. Before you get too excited and blend along, you must remember that great care must be exercised during the processing and of the foods above so as to not destroy their mineral contents. There are also things you have to remember to maximize the benefits of your green smoothies. Below are some tips to ensure you get the full benefits of your smoothie:

Tip #1: Invest on a high quality blender.

If your blender takes at least 2 minutes to produce a nice, even consistency for your smoothie, then you definitely need to buy another one. Blending should generally take only a maximum of 40 seconds to prevent heat from destroying valuable enzymes. Blending should also consist of short pulses to prevent heat build-up.

Tip #2: Slice the ingredients first into smaller pieces.

Do this especially for hard, fibrous fruits and vegetables as this will greatly reduce the blending time.

Tip #3: Place the juiciest ingredients at the bottom of the blender.

This practice will create more liquid so it will be easier to liquefy harder and more fibrous vegetables.

Tip #4: Never hesitate to add water or any other thinner if you feel it is necessary.

Adding water or thinners will lubricate the ingredients averting too much friction and heat build-up. The more liquid there is initially, the faster the blender can liquefy other ingredients. If you are concerned with thinning of the flavor, you can add more fruits or vegetables. Do not hesitate to experiment.

Tip #5: Drink your smoothie as soon as possible.

Too long exposure to the air can degrade the nutrient content of your smoothies. Of course, as much as possible we want to maximize the health benefits of green smoothies, it is inherent that some of the nutrients will be lost during processing. In fact, degradation starts right after severing a fruit's connection to the plant during harvest. The mere act of biting, slicing, processing and even chewing of these fruits and vegetables trigger some oxidation.

Do not be depressed as this is normal, this may actually be the rationale why we need to eat our vegetables everyday! Anyway, the point is, degradation should happen inside your gut, and not anywhere else that is why drinking your smoothie as soon as possible is important. In the event that this is impossible, put your smoothie inside a dark container and refrigerate it. Smoothies stored this way must be consumed within 48 hours.

Tip #6: Try to add in-season vegetables in your smoothies.

This practice will not only be infinitely cheaper, this will also broaden your range of nutrient intake. Never be afraid to add vegetables that you have not tasted before. In striving for a complete nutrition, variety is the key.

Tip #7: Research on the foods you eat.

You are what you eat, the cliché goes. Knowing more about what you put inside your body will help you make more informed decisions. As said earlier, everything we think we know about food is in chaos. Every year, new scientific facts about "healthy foods" and "bad foods" are being unraveled so you have to be vigilant. Simply knowing the nutrient content of that hated vegetable of yours may give you some spark of enthusiasm so you can eat it with a happy face.

CHAPTER 4- THE BENEFITS OF GREEN SMOOTHIE CLEANSE

You have seen from the previous chapter that what makes a green smoothie special and ideal for cleansing are the right ingredients. For example the pro-digestive properties of ginger together with fiber and probiotics can improve digestive function, priming your digestive system for more efficient nutrient absorption. Coupled with the fact that the ingredients are blended together, absorption, assimilation and distribution of the nutrients to all your cells will take little time.

The antioxidants like vitamins A, C and E will remove free radicals from your cells that are associated with premature aging. The anticancer agents may help prevent the development of abnormal cells associated with cancer. The fact that cleansing will take place along a particular time period means that your body will always be supplied by these nutrients. That is why, theoretically, after cleansing, you will feel rejuvenated and ready to take on the stress and pollution of the world.

If you do not have time to spare on a cleansing period,

sipping on green smoothies once in a while will do you so much favor. Of course, it will not have the same rejuvenating effect than when you undergo cleansing but this healthy beverage will definitely have its place in your life. Here are the many benefits offered by green smoothies outside cleansing:

- **Keeps you hydrated!**

This is most important during summer and for people who are trying to lose weight. Although you are not technically drinking pure water, your body is designed to also get water from foods and beverages that you eat and drink. Keeping hydrated will not only contribute to a feeling of satiety so you have less chance to overeat but also make your metabolism faster, increasing your body's capacity to burn fat.

- **You can drink green smoothies for breakfast!**

As long as your green smoothie has adequate fat, fiber and protein to keep you sated, drinking green smoothies during breakfast is a great way to replenish the lost energy and nutrients spent by your body during sleep and to power you throughout the day. A green smoothie is also a perfect breakfast for those who are on the go as it takes very little time and effort to prepare. Even clean-up is a breeze since all you need is your blender and your glass.

- **You can share the joy and benefits of smoothies with the rest of your family!**

This is especially true for children. It is a way for you to make sure your children are getting their needed vitamins and minerals to grow without threatening or begging them. It also teaches them the importance of watching what they eat at a very early age.

- **Drink smoothies before/after exercise for energy boost!**

Since the nutrient content of green smoothies are complete and can be easily assimilated, you can drink smoothies to replenish lost ions (especially if you use coconut water) and energy as well as supply the body with the needed proteins to build bigger muscles (add a lot of protein to your smoothie). For those who want to get in shape through exercise and cutting down on food intake, green smoothies can serve as one-bowl meals that unlike juices, can still provide enough energy and proteins to continue body functions.

A FINAL WORD

Smoothies should be included on anyone's diet, since they are really beneficial to anyone's health. You can easily prepare this drink without hassle; you do not need so much time making your own smoothie. Aside from that, the ingredients that you will need does not cost that much.

If you are ready to experience all of the amazing benefits of consuming green smoothies, go out and purchase some of your favorite organic fruits and greens and give it a try. It is actually fun to come up with different mixtures of fruits and greens, and you cannot go wrong. As long as you like the flavor of the fruit you are using, you are sure to enjoy the taste of your smoothie. These smoothies truly are the fastest and easiest way to obtain a healthier lifestyle.

Please Leave a Review

Finally, if you enjoyed this book, please take the time to share your thoughts and post a review on Amazon. It would be greatly appreciated.

That review and feedback will help me improve the content in my books – and make each and every one more relevant and helpful to you.

Thank you again and good luck!

J.C. Collins